THE NEW PREPPER WATER PURIFICATION SURVIVAL GUIDE

Learn how to find, filter, purify water for survival and emergency preparedness with step by step instructions

JEFF GOODMAN

Introduction

In a world where preparedness is key to facing unforeseen challenges, one element stands out as an absolute necessity: water. Welcome to "The New Prepper Water Purification Survival Guide," your comprehensive resource for navigating the critical realm of water purification in prepping.

Brief Overview of the Importance of Water Purification in Prepping: Water is life, and in a prepper's toolkit, ensuring a clean and sustainable water supply is paramount. Chapter II delves into understanding water sources, guiding you through identifying potential sources and assessing the risks of contamination. It lays the foundation for a resilient water strategy in any survival scenario.

Purpose of the Guide: This guide is more than just a manual; it's a roadmap to mastering the art of water purification for preppers. From essential methods like boiling, filtration, and chemical purification (Chapter III) to hands-on, do-it-yourself solutions explored in Chapter IV, you'll gain practical insights that transcend theory.

As we venture into water storage strategies (Chapter V) and explore emergency water sources (Chapter VI), you'll be equipped to adapt to various situations. The guide doesn't just stop at methods; it helps you choose the right tools (Chapter VII) and develop a customized plan (Chapter VIII) based on your unique location and resources.

Real-world applications come to life in Chapter IX, where case studies and success stories illustrate effective water purification in survival situations. But, it's not just about successes – Chapter X addresses troubleshooting and common mistakes, ensuring you learn from challenges others have faced.

Safety and health considerations take center stage in Chapter XI, emphasizing the importance of ensuring water safety for consumption and understanding the health risks associated with contaminated water.

Embark on this journey through "The New Prepper Water Purification Survival Guide," where each chapter is a stepping stone towards water security, a fundamental element in your preparedness arsenal. Let's navigate these waters together, ensuring you're not just surviving, but thriving in any circumstance.

Chapter II: Understanding Water Sources

A. Identifying Potential Water Sources: In the intricate dance of survival, the first step is to recognize the stage – and when it comes to water, knowing where to find it is pivotal. This chapter is your guide to identifying potential water sources in a prepper's landscape.

Natural Sources:

Rivers, lakes, and streams: Understanding the dynamics of flowing water and the potential risks associated with these sources.

Springs: Identifying natural springs and evaluating their reliability as a consistent water source.

Groundwater: Exploring the possibilities of accessing water from wells and underground aquifers.

Urban and Built Environments:

Rainwater harvesting: Unveiling the potential of rain as a valuable water source and methods to collect and store it.

Urban infrastructure: Tapping into city water supplies, recognizing the challenges, and optimizing usage in an urban setting.

Unconventional Sources:
Plant-based sources: Recognizing certain plants that can provide water and understanding how to extract it safely.

Human-made structures: Investigating unconventional sources like abandoned buildings or man-made reservoirs.

B. Assessing Water Quality and Contamination Risks: Identifying a water source is just the beginning; understanding its quality and potential risks is the key to ensuring a safe water supply for prepping.

Visual Inspection:

Color and clarity: Analyzing the visual aspects of water to detect visible contaminants.

Odor: Recognizing unusual smells that may indicate contamination.

Testing Methods:
Water testing kits: Exploring the use of readily available kits to assess water quality on-site.

Simple testing techniques: Learning DIY methods to gauge water purity in a resource-constrained environment.

Common Contaminants:
Bacteria, viruses, and parasites: Understanding the health risks associated with biological contaminants.

Chemical pollutants: Identifying and addressing potential chemical hazards in water sources.

Environmental Factors:
Industrial areas and pollution: Recognizing the impact of industrial activities on water quality.

Natural contaminants: Dealing with issues like sedimentation and mineral content in specific environments.

Remember, "in the realm of water purification, knowledge is the compass guiding you toward a reliable and safe water supply for your prepping endeavors".

Chapter III: Essential Water Purification Methods

A. Boiling Techniques and Precautions: In the crucible of survival, boiling stands as one of the oldest and most reliable methods to render water safe for consumption. This chapter unveils the art of boiling, offering not just a technique but a mastery of the process.

Proper Boiling Procedures:

Duration and intensity: Understanding the optimal boiling time and temperature for effective pathogen elimination.

Boiling in various settings: Adapting the boiling method to different situations, whether indoors or outdoors.

Contaminant Elimination:

Bacteria, viruses, and parasites: Delving into how boiling eradicates microbial threats.

Chemical contaminants: Assessing the effectiveness of boiling in removing certain chemical pollutants.

Precautions and Considerations:

Conserving fuel: Maximizing the efficiency of boiling in resource-limited scenarios.

Safe handling: Tips for safely handling hot water and preventing burns or injuries.

B. Filtration Systems and Options: When the waters run murky, filtration emerges as a vital tool. This section guides you through the intricate world of filtration systems, ensuring your water is not only clear but also safe.

Types of Filtration Systems:

Portable filters: Exploring options suitable for preppers on the move.

Gravity filters: Understanding their efficiency in larger quantities of water.

DIY filtration methods: Crafting filters from readily available materials in emergency situations.

Filtering Contaminants:

Size-specific filtration: Addressing different contaminants based on their particle size.

Activated carbon filters: Utilizing these filters to trap chemicals and improve water taste.

Maintenance and Longevity:

Cleaning and replacing filters: Ensuring the longevity and effectiveness of your filtration system.

Storage considerations: Tips for storing filters to prevent contamination when not in use.

C. Chemical Purification Methods: In the toolkit of prepper water purification, chemicals play a strategic role. This section explores the nuances of chemical purification, providing a comprehensive understanding of its applications.

Common Purification Chemicals:

Chlorine and iodine: Assessing their effectiveness in disinfection and their respective pros and cons.

Water purification tablets: Exploring convenient, pre-packaged solutions for chemical treatment.

Dosage and Contact Time:

Ensuring proper chemical concentration: Calculating and applying the right amount for effective purification.

Understanding contact time: Allowing chemicals sufficient time to neutralize contaminants.

Limitations and Considerations:

Chemical taste and odor: Addressing potential drawbacks and ways to mitigate undesirable effects.

Storage stability: Maintaining the potency of purification chemicals over time.

Armed with the knowledge from this chapter, you'll possess a diversified arsenal of water purification methods, ready to adapt to any circumstance that may arise in your prepping journey.

Chapter IV: DIY Water Purification Solutions

A. Building Homemade Water Filters: In the realm of prepper ingenuity, crafting your own water filters can be a game-changer. This chapter is a hands-on guide to building effective homemade filters using easily accessible materials.

Materials and Components:

Exploring common household items: Identifying materials like gravel, sand, and activated charcoal for filtration.

Improvised filter containers: Using everyday objects like plastic bottles or containers as the framework for your homemade filter.

Step-by-Step Construction:

Layering for filtration: Understanding the sequence of materials to optimize particle removal.

Securing the filter: Ensuring stability and durability in various environments.

Adaptability and Portability:

Tailoring filters to specific needs: Adapting designs for different water sources and contaminant types.

Creating compact, portable filters: Ideal for preppers on the move or in emergency scenarios.

B. Creating Improvised Purification Devices: When resources are scarce, preppers rely on creativity. This section explores the art of crafting improvised purification devices, ensuring water safety with minimal resources.

Solar Still Construction:

Harnessing solar power: Building a solar still to collect and purify water using natural energy.

Simple materials: Utilizing basic materials like plastic sheeting and containers for construction.

Improvised Distillation Methods:

DIY distillation apparatus: Creating a makeshift distillation setup for purifying water through evaporation and condensation.

Heat sources: Exploring alternative heat sources for distillation in different scenarios.

Emergency Water Filtration Tools:

Emergency straw filters: Crafting a simple yet effective straw filter for on-the-go water purification.

Cloth filtration methods: Using readily available fabrics for quick filtration in emergency situations.

Field-Tested DIY Solutions:

Real-world examples: Showcasing success stories of preppers who effectively utilized DIY water purification methods.

By the end of this chapter, you'll not only have the knowledge to construct your own water filters and purification devices but also the confidence to adapt and innovate in the face of challenging circumstances. Embrace the DIY spirit, and empower yourself with practical skills for water purification in any prepper scenario

Chapter V: Water Storage Strategies

A. Proper Container Selection and Maintenance:
Effective water storage is not only about having the right quantity but also about ensuring the water remains safe for consumption. This chapter delves into the intricacies of selecting appropriate containers and maintaining them for long-term water storage.

Container Materials:

Plastic, glass, and metal containers: Assessing the pros and cons of each material for durability and safety.

Food-grade considerations: Understanding the importance of using containers designed for safe water storage.

Sealing and Lid Security:
Air-tight seals: Ensuring lids create a secure barrier to prevent contamination.

UV protection: Shielding water from sunlight to avoid algae growth and degradation of container materials.

Regular Inspection and Cleaning:

Mold and residue prevention: Implementing routines to inspect and clean containers to maintain water quality.

Repairing damages: Addressing cracks or leaks promptly to prevent water loss and contamination.

B. Long-Term Water Storage Considerations:
Prepping is about looking ahead, and long-term water storage is a critical aspect of that foresight. This section explores the factors to consider when storing water for extended periods.

Water Rotation Strategies:
Regular usage and replacement: Creating a rotation schedule to use and replenish stored water.

Monitoring expiration dates: Checking and adhering to expiration dates of water stored in commercially bottled containers.

Preservatives and Stabilizers:
Adding chlorine or hydrogen peroxide: Exploring methods to extend the shelf life of stored water.

Oxygen absorbers: Using these to reduce oxidation and maintain water quality over time.

Temperature and Location:
Avoiding extreme temperatures: Placing water storage containers in cool, dark areas to prevent heat-induced deterioration.

Elevating containers: Minimizing the risk of contamination by keeping stored water off the ground.

Scaling Up Storage for Groups:
Community prepping: Considering water storage solutions for larger groups or families.

Water distribution systems: Exploring ways to efficiently manage and share stored water resources.

By the end of this chapter, you'll possess the knowledge to not only choose the right containers for water storage but also implement effective maintenance and long-term storage strategies. Water security is not just about what you have today but ensuring a sustainable and reliable supply for the challenges that tomorrow may bring.

Chapter VI: Emergency Water Sources

A. Rainwater Harvesting: In the intricate dance of survival, rainwater emerges as a natural and replenishable source. This chapter delves into the art of rainwater harvesting, offering preppers a valuable technique for sourcing water in times of need.

Collection Systems:

Roof catchment systems: Designing effective systems to collect rainwater from rooftops.

Gutter and downspout setups: Optimizing rainwater flow into storage containers.

Water Quality Considerations:

Initial runoff: Addressing potential contaminants on roofs and ensuring the first flush of rainwater is diverted.

Filtration methods: Employing filters to enhance the quality of harvested rainwater.

Storage Solutions:

Rain barrels and cisterns: Selecting and installing containers suitable for storing harvested rainwater.

Integration with existing systems: Incorporating rainwater harvesting into your overall water storage strategy.

B. Extracting Water from Unconventional Sources:
Survival often demands thinking outside the norm, and water extraction from unconventional sources can be a lifeline. This section explores innovative methods to secure water when conventional sources are scarce.

Moisture Condensation Techniques:

Solar stills: Constructing solar-powered stills to extract water from moist soil or vegetation.

Improvised condensation traps: Utilizing available materials to create simple yet effective condensation systems.

Transpiration Bags and Plant Sources:

Transpiration bag usage: Tapping into trees for a slow but steady source of water.

Edible plant water content: Identifying plants with high water content for potential extraction.

Human-Made Reservoirs and Structures:
Utilizing abandoned structures: Extracting water from neglected buildings or infrastructure.

Water extraction from vehicles: Safely accessing water from abandoned or non-functional vehicles.

Purification of Unconventional Sources:

Assessing contamination risks: Understanding potential hazards in unconventional water sources.

Applying purification methods: Using previously discussed techniques to ensure extracted water is safe for consumption.

By the end of this chapter, you'll be equipped with the knowledge and skills to harness rainwater efficiently and extract water from unconventional sources when faced with emergency scenarios.

Chapter VII: Choosing the Right Purification Tools

A. Evaluating Water Purification Tablets and Drops:
In the toolkit of a prepper, the choice of purification tablets and drops can be a swift and efficient means to ensure water safety. This chapter dives into the nuances of these chemical solutions, providing a comprehensive guide for evaluation.

Types of Purification Chemicals:

Chlorine tablets: Assessing the effectiveness and versatility of chlorine-based tablets.

Iodine tablets and drops: Understanding their applications and considering potential drawbacks.

Dosage and Contact Time:

Proper chemical concentration: Calculating the right amount of purification chemicals for varying water conditions.

Contact time considerations: Allowing sufficient time for tablets or drops to work before consuming the water.

Storage and Shelf Life:

Stability of chemicals: Ensuring the potency of purification tablets and drops over extended periods.

Storage conditions: Ideal environments to maintain the effectiveness of chemical purification tools.

B. Selecting Portable Water Purifiers: When mobility is crucial, portable water purifiers become indispensable. This section guides preppers through the process of choosing the right purifiers to match their needs and circumstances.

Filtration Mechanisms:
Pump filters: Evaluating hand-pumped systems for their efficiency in removing contaminants.

Squeeze and gravity filters: Exploring alternative methods for portable, on-the-go filtration.

Filter Pore Size and Micron Ratings:
Understanding the significance of pore size: Selecting filters based on the specific contaminants you aim to remove.

Micron ratings: Interpreting filter specifications for optimal purification results.

Flow Rate and Capacity:
Considering water output: Assessing the speed at which different purifiers can deliver clean water.

Capacity for group use: Choosing purifiers that meet the demands of a larger prepping community.

Durability and Maintenance:
Construction materials: Evaluating the durability of purifier components for longevity.

Ease of cleaning: Selecting purifiers that are simple to maintain in the field.

These tools are the frontline defense in ensuring a safe water supply during your prepping journey, and understanding their strengths and limitations is vital for effective water purification.

Chapter VIII: Developing a Water Purification Plan

A. Customizing a Plan Based on Location and Resources: One size doesn't fit all in the world of prepping, and your water purification plan should be no exception. This chapter emphasizes the importance of tailoring your strategy to the specific characteristics of your location and the resources at your disposal.

Geographical Considerations:
Urban vs. rural environments: Adapting purification techniques to suit the unique challenges of different settings.

Climate influences: Recognizing the impact of weather patterns on water availability and contamination risks.

Local Water Sources:
Mapping water resources: Identifying nearby natural water sources and understanding their quality.

Navigating legal restrictions: Complying with local regulations governing water collection and purification.

Resource Assessment:
Equipment availability: Evaluating the tools and materials you have on hand for water purification.

Community collaboration: Leveraging local networks to share resources and expertise.

B. Training on Purification Techniques: Knowledge is your most valuable asset in the realm of prepper water purification. This section emphasizes the necessity of ongoing education and training to hone your skills.

Hands-On Training:
Practical exercises: Simulating water purification scenarios to reinforce theoretical knowledge.

Group training sessions: Learning from and sharing experiences with fellow preppers.

Utilizing Educational Resources:
Online guides and videos: Tapping into digital resources for continuous learning and skill development.

Books and manuals: Building a reference library to deepen your understanding of water purification techniques.

Mock Scenarios and Drills:
Emergency simulations: Replicating real-world scenarios
to test the efficiency of your purification plan.

Regular drills: Maintaining a state of readiness through
routine practices.

Seeking Expert Guidance:
Collaborating with experts: Engaging with professionals
in the field of water purification for specialized insights.

Participating in workshops: Attending events or
workshops to learn from experienced practitioners.

By the end of this chapter, you'll have the tools to design
a water purification plan tailored to your unique
circumstances and the knowledge to continually refine
and enhance your skills through ongoing training.
Preparing for water-related challenges isn't just a
one-time effort – it's a dynamic process that evolves with
your understanding and the changing conditions of your
environment.

Chapter IX: Case Studies and Success Stories

A. Real-Life Examples of Effective Water Purification in Survival Situations: This chapter delves into the experiences of preppers who have successfully navigated challenging situations, showcasing real-life examples of effective water purification. These stories serve as beacons of inspiration and practical insights for fellow preppers.

Remote Wilderness Survival:
Narratives of preppers stranded in remote locations and their ingenious water purification solutions.

Strategies for sourcing and purifying water in the wild without conventional tools.

Urban Prepping:
Testimonials from individuals who faced water scarcity in urban environments and triumphed through strategic planning.

Urban-specific purification techniques and adaptations based on case studies.

Natural Disaster Preparedness:
Accounts from preppers who successfully managed
water needs during and after natural disasters.

The role of quick decision-making and improvisation in
challenging circumstances.

B. Lessons Learned and Practical Tips: Beyond the
narratives, this section distills the wisdom gained from
these case studies into practical lessons and tips for
preppers to enhance their own water purification
strategies.

Adaptability in Methods:
Learning to adapt purification methods based on the
specific challenges faced in different survival scenarios.

Flexibility in approach and the importance of having a
diverse set of skills.

Community Collaboration:
Examples of successful community efforts in sourcing,
purifying, and distributing water.

The power of collaboration in overcoming water-related
challenges in group settings.

Effective Resource Utilization:

Insights into how preppers efficiently utilized available resources for water purification.

Making the most of limited tools and materials in emergency situations.

Continuous Improvement:
Testimonials reflecting the evolution of preppers' water purification plans over time.

The significance of learning from both successes and challenges to refine strategies.

Mental Preparedness:
Personal reflections on the psychological aspects of facing water-related emergencies.

Maintaining a resilient mindset and adapting to unforeseen circumstances.

By the end of this chapter, readers will gain a profound understanding of the practical applications of water purification strategies through the shared experiences of real-life preppers. The lessons learned and practical tips will serve as valuable insights, enriching your own prepping journey and fostering a sense of community resilience.

Chapter X: Troubleshooting and Common Mistakes

A. Addressing Challenges in Purification Processes:
This chapter serves as a guide for preppers to navigate and overcome challenges encountered during water purification processes. Recognizing and addressing these issues ensures a more resilient and effective water purification strategy.

Inadequate Filtration:
Identifying common filtration problems, such as clogging or improper setup.

Troubleshooting techniques to optimize filtration systems for consistent performance.

Insufficient Boiling:
Addressing issues related to inadequate heat sources or improper boiling techniques.

Tips for optimizing boiling processes to ensure complete pathogen elimination.

Chemical Purification Concerns:
Troubleshooting situations where chemical purification
methods may fall short.
Adjusting dosage and contact time to address specific
challenges.

B. Avoiding Pitfalls in Prepper Water Preparation:
Preparedness is a proactive endeavor, but it's crucial to
steer clear of common pitfalls that can undermine your
water purification efforts. This section outlines potential
mistakes and provides insights to avoid them.

Lack of Regular Maintenance:
Highlighting the importance of routinely inspecting and
cleaning water storage containers and purification tools.

Preventive measures to ensure the longevity and
efficiency of equipment.

Overlooking Environmental Factors:
Recognizing how climate, temperature, and local
conditions can impact water storage and purification.

Strategies to adapt to changing environmental
circumstances.

Ignoring Local Regulations:
Emphasizing the necessity of understanding and complying with local laws regarding water collection and purification.

Consequences of neglecting legal considerations in prepper water preparation.

Failure to Rotate Stored Water:
Addressing the risks associated with storing water for extended periods without regular rotation.

Developing a practical schedule for using and replenishing stored water.

Overreliance on a Single Method:
Discussing the dangers of depending solely on one purification method.
Strategies for diversifying your approach to enhance overall water security.
By delving into troubleshooting and highlighting common mistakes, this chapter aims to fortify your water purification plan against potential setbacks. Learning from challenges and avoiding pitfalls ensures that your prepping efforts are resilient, adaptable, well-prepared to navigate the uncertainties of survival scenarios.

Chapter XI: Safety and Health Considerations

A. Ensuring Water Safety for Consumption: This chapter is dedicated to the paramount importance of maintaining water safety for consumption. Preppers must prioritize not only securing water but ensuring that it poses no health risks when consumed.

Microbial Contamination:
Health Risks: Explore the specific health risks associated with various microbial contaminants found in untreated water, ranging from gastrointestinal issues to more severe diseases.

Purification Methods: Delve into the effectiveness of different purification methods such as boiling, filtration, and chemical treatments in eliminating or reducing microbial threats.

Chemical Contaminants:
Identifying Hazards: Provide a comprehensive list of potential chemical pollutants that can be present in water sources, including industrial runoff, heavy metals, and agricultural chemicals.

Purification Strategies: Detail purification methods tailored to neutralizing specific chemical contaminants, emphasizing the importance of choosing methods based on the water's chemical composition.

Biological Hazards:
Risk Factors: Examine the risks associated with biological contaminants like algae and fungi, including allergic reactions and other health implications.

Preventive Measures: Offer strategies for preventing and treating waterborne biological hazards, incorporating both purification methods and proactive measures during water collection.

Safe Water Storage Practices:
Container Selection: Provide guidance on selecting appropriate containers for water storage, considering factors like material, size, and seal integrity.

Hygiene Maintenance: Stress the importance of maintaining a clean and hygienic storage environment to prevent secondary contamination of stored water.

B. Health Risks Associated with Contaminated Water:

Waterborne Diseases: Common Diseases: Detail the symptoms, treatment, and preventive measures for prevalent waterborne diseases such as cholera, dysentery, and giardiasis.

Geographical Considerations: Discuss how the prevalence of certain diseases may vary based on geographical locations and environmental conditions.

Long-Term Health Effects:
Cumulative Impact: Explore the potential cumulative health effects of prolonged exposure to certain water contaminants, emphasizing the need for consistent water safety practices.

Chronic Health Risks: Highlight chronic health risks associated with consuming contaminated water over extended periods, including organ damage and developmental issues.

Vulnerable Populations:
Special Considerations: Offer tailored water safety measures for vulnerable populations, recognizing the increased susceptibility of children, the elderly, and those with compromised immune systems.

Caregiver Guidelines: Provide guidance for caregivers and preppers responsible for vulnerable individuals, emphasizing additional precautions.

Mental Health Considerations: Psychological Impact: Discuss the potential psychological impact of water-related health concerns, including anxiety and stress.

Coping Strategies: Provide strategies for maintaining mental well-being during challenging circumstances, emphasizing the importance of a holistic approach to health and preparedness.

By thoroughly exploring these subtopics, preppers will gain a nuanced understanding of the complexities involved in ensuring water safety for consumption and mitigating health risks associated with contaminated water. This knowledge forms a robust foundation for creating effective and sustainable water purification plans in various prepping scenarios.

Chapter XII: Conclusion - Prioritizing Water Purification in Prepping

In concluding "The New Prepper Water Purification Survival Guide," let's recap key points and emphasize the critical importance of prioritizing water purification in your prepping endeavors.

A. Recap of Key Points:

Understanding Water Sources:
Identifying potential water sources, assessing quality, and recognizing the diverse nature of water in different environments.

Essential Water Purification Methods:
Mastering boiling techniques, filtration systems, and chemical purification methods to ensure a versatile toolkit for water safety.

DIY Water Purification Solutions:
Building homemade filters and crafting improvised purification devices, showcasing the power of adaptability in resource-limited scenarios.

Water Storage Strategies: Proper container selection, long-term considerations, and the importance of rotational practices to maintain a consistent and safe water supply.

Emergency Water Sources:
Harnessing rainwater and extracting water from unconventional sources, showcasing resilience in the face of unforeseen circumstances.

Choosing the Right Purification Tools:
Evaluating water purification tablets and drops, selecting portable purifiers, and understanding the strengths and limitations of each tool.

Developing a Water Purification Plan:
Customizing plans based on location and resources, coupled with ongoing training to refine and enhance purification skills.

Case Studies and Success Stories:
Real-life examples providing inspiration and practical insights, accompanied by lessons learned and practical tips from those who have navigated water-related challenges.

Troubleshooting and Common Mistakes:
Addressing challenges in purification processes and avoiding pitfalls to maintain a robust and resilient water purification strategy.

Safety and Health Considerations:
Ensuring water safety for consumption, understanding health risks, and implementing measures to safeguard both physical and mental well-being.

B. Encouragement for Readers to Prioritize Water Purification:

As you embark on your prepping journey, remember that water is the essence of survival. It's not merely a commodity; it's the lifeline that sustains us through the unforeseen challenges that life may throw our way. The knowledge you've gained in this guide empowers you to be the steward of your water security, ensuring that you and your loved ones have a continuous and safe supply.

In the realm of prepping, water purification is a cornerstone. It's not just a task to check off a list; it's a continuous commitment to preparedness, adaptability, and resilience. Prioritize water purification, not as a reactive measure, but as an integral part of your proactive strategy for any eventuality.

Water is not only a physical necessity but a symbol of life's continuity. As you safeguard your water supply, you're not just preparing for survival; you're embracing a lifestyle that values self-sufficiency, community collaboration, and the unwavering spirit of a true prepper.

Remember, in the face of uncertainty, a well-prepared prepper stands firm with the knowledge, skills, and resources to overcome challenges. The journey doesn't end here; it's an ongoing commitment to learning, adapting, and thriving. May your water purification efforts be a beacon of resilience in your prepping endeavors.

Stay prepared, stay safe, and may your path be clear, and your water always pure.